CODY SMITH

8 Weeks to 200 Consecutive Sit-ups

Build a Strong Core by Working Your Abs, Obliques, and Lower Back | at Home Workouts | No Gym Required |

First edition

ISBN: 978-1-952381-15-7

This book was professionally typeset on Reedsy.
Find out more at reedsy.com

Contents

Before You Begin

Hey reader, thanks for grabbing a copy of the book.

If you are looking to pair this workout program with a complimentary guide to shed weight and boost your growth hormones to build more muscle faster, then I've got you covered.

Seems crazy to do both at the same time, but you can.

Better still, it is stupid easy.

Oh, and it is free. You can do this method anytime you want, anywhere for the rest of your life.

I usually sell this information, but I want you to have it.

You can get a copy from your cell phone from a simple text.

Seriously, get your phone out and text BOOST to (678) 506-7543.

Cheers!

Introduction - How to Use This Book

If you asked random people on the street how to get six pack abs, they would probably tell you to do crunches.

Sure, they work your abs but not like sit-ups.

Sit-ups work your entire core when done correctly, but you would see a whole lot of people doing them in the gym.

You will find people working on workout equipment for hours when all they need is their body to get the job done.

And you would be hard pressed to find a lot of people even in a gym who can do even 50 consecutive sit-ups.

But we are not here to shoot for a mere 50. We are going straight for 200 consecutive smackeroos.

We are hitting 3 digits here or we are going home. All or nothing baby.

And that's exactly what you're going to find here in this 8-week program.

Sure, you could do sit-ups on your own, try and knock out as many as possible every day and work your way to 200 but you are either going to fall short or give up before you even get there.

What you need is strategically designed workouts for your current fitness level that challenge you just enough without killing you. Each workout will push you for the proper progression to make steady gains along the way. This program is structured to take all the guesswork out of your journey to 200 consecutive sit-ups.

And these workouts that can literally be completed anywhere as long as you have somewhere, something, or someone to anchor your feet.

Your journey begins with an initial sit-up assessment to find out where your current max is. Afterwards, you will know exactly where to start in the program.

Once you complete the entire program, you will have earned the right to attempt nailing 200 consecutive sit-ups.

Some people knock it out on their first try. Others will not and will need to hack it a few more weeks before trying again.

Now, I will warn you, these workouts can feel very repetitive at times. Far too often people look for variety and complexity to see results when really the simplest of approaches is best.

100 sit-ups variations and off the wall workout routines are not what is going to get you to the results you want. Showing up and putting in the work; that is where the real bacon is.

Some of you will not need the entire 8 weeks. Others will need more than 8 weeks. Either way is perfectly fine and doesn't mean the program doesn't work, it just means everyone comes from a different level of fitness.

8 weeks is not some magical number that will work for every single person. 8 weeks is the average amount of time it will take the average person to reach 200 consecutive sit-ups so do not get too caught up in the timeline. It will take you however long that it takes you.

What I can promise you is if you put in the work, you will see the results.

Up next is the initial assessment. Get after it, champ.

Initial Sit-up Assessment

This is the first step into your incredible journey to doing 200 consecutive sit-ups. It will be hard but manageable as you embark on something that very few people on the face of the earth have ever accomplished.

We are going to start out with a sit-up assessment to determine where you should start in the program.

Make sure you are doing full sit-ups going all the way through the motion. Proper form is key to getting the most out of this exercise, so I'll quickly go over how to properly perform a sit-up.

Lie on your back with knees bent at 90 degrees with your feet anchored. Tuck your chin into your neck or chest as you either interlace your fingers at the base of your skull or place both hands on the opposite upper chest/shoulder area. You will begin the exercise by lifting your upper body toward your thighs until your upper body is roughly perpendicular to the ground. Slowly lower your upper body back down to the floor to point where your shoulder blades touch the ground before raising your upper body back up to complete the next rep.

It is important that you do not use your arms or heads to thrust your upper body toward your thighs. This is just cheating yourself out of doing a correct sit-up. All reps should be performed in a controlled manner.

Go ahead and complete as many correct sit-ups as you can without stopping using something sturdy to anchor your feet like a toe bar, couch, or dresser.

Once you are done, remember the number of fully completed sit-ups and head to the post assessment results section.

Note: If this is the first assessment, you will write your assessment number in the '1st assessment' row. When you come back to do another assessment, you write in your completed number of reps in the respective row depending on how many assessments you have completed.

_____ reps: 1st assessment

_____ reps: 2nd assessment

_____ reps: 3rd assessment

_____ reps: 4th assessment

_____ reps: 5th assessment

_____ reps: 6th assessment

_____ reps: 7th assessment

_____ reps: 8th assessment

_____ reps: 9th assessment

_____ reps: 10th assessment

_____ reps: 11th assessment

_____ reps: 12th assessment

_____ reps: 13th assessment

_____ reps: 14th assessment

_____ reps: 15th assessment

_____ reps: 16th assessment

_____ reps: 17th assessment

_____ reps: 18th assessment

_____ reps: 19th assessment

_____ reps: 20th assessment

Post-Assessment Results

So... how did you do?

Were you surprised with how many you did or were you underwhelmed and disappointed that you did not do so hot?

Do not beat yourself up. This is simply a baseline for you to start from.

Go ahead and jog your memory of your assessment score.

With that score in mind, you are now going to be directed to your workout grouping based on your score.

Do not get too caught up in the name of each group of workouts, these are just fun names to identify which group you are currently in. If you do not like your current group name, do not worry, stick with the program long enough and you will be out of that group in no time and into another group whose name you probably will not like either.

Before I go into informing you of your baseline workout, I recommend leaving a day between now and hitting your first workout to recover from your assessment. However, you do not have to if you are feeling gung-ho and want to go ahead and knock out your first workout.

- If you did less than 10, you will start in the foundations group to build up your strength.
- If you did 10, you will start in the Novice Group.
- If you did between 11 and 20, you will start in the Newb Group.
- If you did between 21 and 30, you will start in the Greenhorn Group.
- If you did between 31 and 40, you will start in the Cub Group.
- If you did between 41 and 50, you will start in the Rookie Group.
- If you did between 51 and 60, you will start in the Pleb Group.
- If you did between 61 and 70, you will start in the Gorilla Group.
- If you did between 71 and 80, you will start in the Viking Group.
- If you did between 81 and 90, you will start in the Elite Group.
- If you did between 91 and 100, you will start in the Commando Group.
- If you did between 101 and 110, you will start in the Veteran Group.
- If you did greater than 110, you will start in the Nuclear Group.

Now that you know your group, you know where you will begin for your next workout.

In your group, you will start with workout 1 followed by workout 2 and 3.

For example, let's say you completed 23 reps and you were going to workout Monday, Wednesday and Friday. That would put you in the Greenhorn Group with workout 1 on Monday, Workout 2 on Wednesday, and workout 3 on Friday.

The following week, you would start with greenhorn Group Workout 4 followed by 5 and 6.

Simple enough.

Also, some of your workouts will involve what I call fundamental sit-ups.

Fundamental sit-ups involve a very slow descend and a normal ascend during the sit-up exercise. These work the full range of muscles throughout the entire sit-ups. Typical sit-ups only provide significant tensions when you raise your body from the floor. These sit-ups make you work during the descent and the rise. You will have either 5 or 10 second descends during your workouts.

For example, if you have a set of 3 fundamental sit-ups with 5 seconds descends, you will start in the up, ready position and lower yourself slowly over a 5 second period to the bottom of the exercise when your shoulder blades touch the floor. You will then pull back up to the starting position like a normal sit-up. As soon as you get to the top of the exercise, you will begin gradually lowering yourself back down over another 5 second period for the second rep followed by the third.

They do not sound bad, but boy do they start to burn quick.

Great job on your assessment and get ready for your first workout.

Workout Completion Checklist

Check off your workouts as you complete them:

_____Foundation Group Workout 1

_____Foundation Group Workout 2

_____Foundation Group Workout 3

_____Foundation Group Workout 4

_____Foundation Group Workout 5

_____Foundation Group Workout 6

_____Novice Group Workout 1

_____Novice Group Workout 2

_____Novice Group Workout 3

_____Novice Group Workout 4

_____Novice Group Workout 5

_____Novice Group Workout 6

_____Newb Group Workout 1

_____Newb Group Workout 2

_____Newb Group Workout 3

_____Newb Group Workout 4

_____Newb Group Workout 5

_____Newb Group Workout 6

_____Greenhorn Group Workout 1

_____Greenhorn Group Workout 2

_____Greenhorn Group Workout 3

_____Greenhorn Group Workout 4

_____Greenhorn Group Workout 5

_____Greenhorn Group Workout 6
_____Cub Group Workout 1
_____Cub Group Workout 2
_____Cub Group Workout 3
_____Cub Group Workout 4
_____Cub Group Workout 5
_____Cub Group Workout 6
_____Rookie Group Workout 1
_____Rookie Group Workout 2
_____Rookie Group Workout 3
_____Rookie Group Workout 4
_____Rookie Group Workout 5
_____Rookie Group Workout 6
_____Pleb Group Workout 1
_____Pleb Group Workout 2
_____Pleb Group Workout 3
_____Pleb Group Workout 4
_____Pleb Group Workout 5
_____Pleb Group Workout 6
_____Gorilla Group Workout 1
_____Gorilla Group Workout 2
_____Gorilla Group Workout 3
_____Gorilla Group Workout 4
_____Gorilla Group Workout 5
_____Gorilla Group Workout 6
_____Viking Group Workout 1
_____Viking Group Workout 2
_____Viking Group Workout 3
_____Viking Group Workout 4
_____Viking Group Workout 5
_____Viking Group Workout 6
_____Elite Group Workout 1
_____Elite Group Workout 2

_____Elite Group Workout 3

_____Elite Group Workout 4

_____Elite Group Workout 5

_____Elite Group Workout 6

_____Commando Group Workout 1

_____Commando Group Workout 2

_____Commando Group Workout 3

_____Commando Group Workout 4

_____Commando Group Workout 5

_____Commando Group Workout 6

_____Veteran Group Workout 1

_____Veteran Group Workout 2

_____Veteran Group Workout 3

_____Veteran Group Workout 4

_____Veteran Group Workout 5

_____Veteran Group Workout 6

_____Nuclear Group Workout 1

_____Nuclear Group Workout 2

_____Nuclear Group Workout 3

_____Nuclear Group Workout 4

_____Nuclear Group Workout 5

_____Nuclear Group Workout 6

_____Attempting 200 Consecutive Sit-ups

_____Completed 200 Consecutive Sit-ups: _____ reps.

Pre & Post Program Measurements

The following measurements are 100% optional and are not required to start or finish the program. I know some people will be curious to know other areas that are positively affected by achieving 200 consecutive sit-ups.

Starting weight: _____

Starting sit-up rep max: _____

Starting timed plank hold max: _____

Ending weight: _____

Ending sit-up rep max: _____

Ending time plank hold max: _____

Foundation Group Workouts

Foundation Group Workout 1

Welcome to the Foundation Group Workout 1.

For this workout, you have 5 sets with 60 seconds of rest between each set consisting of negative sit-ups.

Negative sit-ups simply focus on a slow descent without ascending to the up position. This means as soon as you complete your descent, you can stop and rest.

Go ahead and get into the starting position with your feet anchored in the up, ready position, upper body perpendicular to the floor.

Sets:

1. 1 negative sit-up with a 3 second descend.
2. 1 negative sit-up with a 3 second descend.
3. 1 negative sit-up with a 3 second descend.
4. 1 negative sit-up with a 3 second descend.
5. 1 negative sit-up with a 3 second descend.

If you completed this workout, head to Foundation Group Workout 2 for your next session. If not, stick with this one until you complete it.

Foundation Group Workout 2

Welcome to the Foundation Group Workout 2.

For this workout, you have 5 sets with 60 seconds of rest between each set consisting of negative sit-ups.

Remember to focus on proper form throughout your sets and always start in the up, ready position.

Sets:

1. 1 negative sit-up with a 3 second descend.
2. 1 negative sit-up with a 5 second descend.
3. 1 negative sit-up with a 5 second descend.
4. 1 negative sit-up with a 3 second descend.
5. 1 negative sit-up with a 3 second descend.

If you completed this workout, head to Foundation Group Workout 3 for your next session. If not, stick with this one until you complete it.

Foundation Group Workout 3

Welcome to the Foundation Group Workout 3.

For this workout, you have 5 sets with 60 seconds of rest between each set consisting of negative sit-ups.

Remember to focus on proper form throughout your sets and always start in the up, ready position.

Sets:

1. 1 negative sit-up with a 5 second descend.
2. 1 negative sit-up with a 5 second descend.
3. 1 negative sit-up with a 5 second descend.
4. 1 negative sit-up with a 5 second descend.
5. 1 negative sit-up with a 5 second descend.

If you completed this workout, head to Foundation Group Workout 4 for your next session. If not, stick with this one until you complete it.

Foundation Group Workout 4

Welcome to the Foundation Group Workout 4.

For this workout, you have 5 sets with 60 seconds of rest between each set consisting of negative sit-ups.

Remember to focus on proper form throughout your sets and always start in the up, ready position.

Sets:

1. 1 negative sit-up with a 5 second descend.
2. 1 negative sit-up with a 5 second descend.
3. 1 negative sit-up with a 7 second descend.
4. 1 negative sit-up with a 7 second descend.
5. 1 negative sit-up with a 7 second descend.

If you completed this workout, head to Foundation Group Workout 5 for your next session. If not, stick with this one until you complete it.

Foundation Group Workout 5

Welcome to the Foundation Group Workout 5.

For this workout, you have 5 sets with 60 seconds of rest between each set consisting of negative sit-ups.

Remember to focus on proper form throughout your sets and always start in the up, ready position.

Sets:

1. 1 negative sit-up with a 7 second descend.
2. 1 negative sit-up with a 7 second descend.
3. 1 negative sit-up with a 7 second descend.
4. 1 negative sit-up with a 7 second descend.
5. 1 negative sit-up with a 7 second descend.

If you completed this workout, head to Foundation Group Workout 6 for your next session. If not, stick with this one until you complete it.

Foundation Group Workout 6

Welcome to the Foundation Group Workout 6.

For this workout, you have 5 sets with 60 seconds of rest between each set consisting of negative sit-ups.

Remember to focus on proper form throughout your sets and always start in the up, ready position.

Sets:

1. 1 negative sit-up with a 10 second descend.
2. 1 negative sit-up with a 10 second descend.
3. 1 negative sit-up with a 10 second descend.
4. 1 negative sit-up with a 10 second descend.
5. 1 negative sit-up with a 10 second descend.

Since this is the end of a two-week period, it is time to redo your sit-up assessment to check your progress. Rest a day and give the assessment a go to see which Group you will be in next.

Novice Group Workouts

Novice Group Workout 1

Welcome to the Novice Group Workout 1.

For this workout, you have 6 sets with 60 seconds of rest between each set.

Remember to focus on proper form throughout your sets.

Sets:

1. 5 sit-ups
2. 5 sit-ups
3. 5 sit-ups
4. 5 sit-ups
5. 5 sit-ups
6. 1 fundamental sit-up with a 5 second descend.

If you completed this workout, head to Novice Group Workout 2 for your next session. If not, stick with this one until you complete it.

Glasses of water drank today: 1-2-3-4-5-6-7-8-9-10

Hours of sleep last night: 1-2-3-4-5-6-7-8-9-10

Diet: junk: junk food————semi-healthy————healthy

Novice Group Workout 2

Welcome to the Novice Group Workout 2.

For this workout, you have 6 sets with 60 seconds of rest between each set.

Remember to focus on proper form throughout your sets.

Sets:

1. 7 sit-ups
2. 7 sit-ups
3. 7 sit-ups
4. 7 sit-ups
5. 7 sit-ups
6. 2 fundamental sit-ups with a 5 second descend.

If you completed this workout, head to Novice Group Workout 3 for your next session. If not, stick with this one until you complete it.

Glasses of water drank today: 1-2-3-4-5-6-7-8-9-10

Hours of sleep last night: 1-2-3-4-5-6-7-8-9-10

Diet: junk: junk food—————semi-healthy—————healthy

Novice Group Workout 3

Welcome to the Novice Group Workout 3.

For this workout, you have 6 sets with 90 seconds of rest between each set.

Remember to focus on proper form throughout your sets.

Sets:

1. 8 sit-ups
2. 8 sit-ups
3. 8 sit-ups
4. 8 sit-ups
5. 8 sit-ups
6. Max out: perform as many sit-ups as you can.

Max reps: _____

If you completed this workout, head to Novice Group Workout 4 for your next session. If not, stick with this one until you complete it.

Glasses of water drank today: 1-2-3-4-5-6-7-8-9-10

Hours of sleep last night: 1-2-3-4-5-6-7-8-9-10

Diet: junk: junk food—————semi-healthy—————healthy

Novice Group Workout 4

Welcome to the Novice Group Workout 4.

For this workout, you have 6 sets with 60 seconds of rest between each set.

Remember to focus on proper form throughout your sets.

Sets:

1. 10 sit-ups
2. 10 sit-ups
3. 10 sit-ups
4. 10 sit-ups
5. 10 sit-ups
6. 3 fundamental sit-ups with a 5 second descend.

If you completed this workout, head to Novice Group Workout 5 for your next session. If not, stick with this one until you complete it.

Glasses of water drank today: 1-2-3-4-5-6-7-8-9-10

Hours of sleep last night: 1-2-3-4-5-6-7-8-9-10

Diet: junk: junk food————semi-healthy————healthy

Novice Group Workout 5

Welcome to the Novice Group Workout 5.

For this workout, you have 6 sets with 60 seconds of rest between each set.

Remember to focus on proper form throughout your sets.

Sets:

1. 11 sit-ups
2. 11 sit-ups
3. 11 sit-ups
4. 11 sit-ups
5. 11 sit-ups
6. 3 fundamental sit-ups with a 5 second descend.

If you completed this workout, head to Novice Group Workout 6 for your next session. If not, stick with this one until you complete it.

Glasses of water drank today: 1-2-3-4-5-6-7-8-9-10

Hours of sleep last night: 1-2-3-4-5-6-7-8-9-10

Diet: junk: junk food————semi-healthy————healthy

Novice Group Workout 6

Welcome to the Novice Group Workout 6.

For this workout, you have 6 sets with 90 seconds of rest between each set.

Remember to focus on proper form throughout your sets.

Sets:

1. 14 sit-ups
2. 14 sit-ups
3. 14 sit-ups
4. 14 sit-ups
5. 14 sit-ups
6. Max out: perform as many sit-ups as you can.

Max reps: _____

Since this is the end of a two-week period, it is time to redo your sit-up assessment to check your progress if you fully completed this workout.

Rest a day and give the assessment a go to see which Group you will be in next.

Glasses of water drank today: 1-2-3-4-5-6-7-8-9-10

Hours of sleep last night: 1-2-3-4-5-6-7-8-9-10

Diet: junk: junk food————semi-healthy————healthy

Newb Group Workouts

Newb Group Workout 1

Welcome to the Newb Group Workout 1.

For this workout, you have 6 sets with 60 seconds of rest between each set.

Remember to focus on proper form throughout your sets.

Sets:

1. 11 sit-ups
2. 11 sit-ups
3. 11 sit-ups
4. 11 sit-ups
5. 11 sit-ups
6. 2 fundamental sit-ups with a 5 second descend.

If you completed this workout, head to Newb Group Workout 2 for your next session. If not, stick with this one until you complete it.

Glasses of water drank today: 1-2-3-4-5-6-7-8-9-10

Hours of sleep last night: 1-2-3-4-5-6-7-8-9-10

Diet: junk: junk food————semi-healthy————healthy

Newb Group Workout 2

Welcome to the Newb Group Workout 2.

For this workout, you have 6 sets with 60 seconds of rest between each set.

Remember to focus on proper form throughout your sets.

Sets:

1. 14 sit-ups
2. 14 sit-ups
3. 14 sit-ups
4. 14 sit-ups
5. 14 sit-ups
6. 3 fundamental sit-ups with a 5 second descend.

If you completed this workout, head to Newb Group Workout 3 for your next session. If not, stick with this one until you complete it.

Glasses of water drank today: 1-2-3-4-5-6-7-8-9-10

Hours of sleep last night: 1-2-3-4-5-6-7-8-9-10

Diet: junk: junk food————semi-healthy————healthy

Newb Group Workout 3

Welcome to the Newb Group Workout 3.

For this workout, you have 6 sets with 90 seconds of rest between each set.

Remember to focus on proper form throughout your sets.

Sets:

1. 17 sit-ups
2. 17 sit-ups
3. 17 sit-ups
4. 17 sit-ups
5. 17 sit-ups
6. Max out: perform as many sit-ups as you can.

Max reps: _____

If you completed this workout, head to Newb Group Workout 4 for your next session. If not, stick with this one until you complete it.

Glasses of water drank today: 1-2-3-4-5-6-7-8-9-10

Hours of sleep last night: 1-2-3-4-5-6-7-8-9-10

Diet: junk: junk food—————semi-healthy—————healthy

Newb Group Workout 4

Welcome to the Newb Group Workout 4.

For this workout, you have 6 sets with 60 seconds of rest between each set.

Remember to focus on proper form throughout your sets.

Sets:

1. 19 sit-ups
2. 19 sit-ups
3. 19 sit-ups
4. 19 sit-ups
5. 19 sit-ups
6. 5 fundamental sit-ups with a 5 second descend.

If you completed this workout, head to Newb Group Workout 5 for your next session. If not, stick with this one until you complete it.

Glasses of water drank today: 1-2-3-4-5-6-7-8-9-10

Hours of sleep last night: 1-2-3-4-5-6-7-8-9-10

Diet: junk: junk food—————semi-healthy—————healthy

Newb Group Workout 5

Welcome to the Newb Group Workout 5.

For this workout, you have 6 sets with 60 seconds of rest between each set.

Remember to focus on proper form throughout your sets.

Sets:

1. 21 sit-ups
2. 21 sit-ups
3. 21 sit-ups
4. 21 sit-ups
5. 21 sit-ups
6. 6 fundamental sit-ups with a 5 second descend.

If you completed this workout, head to Newb Group Workout 6 for your next session. If not, stick with this one until you complete it.

Glasses of water drank today: 1-2-3-4-5-6-7-8-9-10

Hours of sleep last night: 1-2-3-4-5-6-7-8-9-10

Diet: junk: junk food—————semi-healthy—————healthy

Newb Group Workout 6

Welcome to the Newb Group Workout 6.

For this workout, you have 6 sets with 90 seconds of rest between each set.

Remember to focus on proper form throughout your sets.

Sets:

1. 23 sit-ups
2. 23 sit-ups
3. 23 sit-ups
4. 23 sit-ups
5. 23 sit-ups
6. Max out: perform as many sit-ups as you can.

Max reps: _____

Since this is the end of a two-week period, it is time to redo your sit-up assessment to check your progress if you fully completed this workout.

Rest a day and give the assessment a go to see which Group you will be in next.

Glasses of water drank today: 1-2-3-4-5-6-7-8-9-10

Hours of sleep last night: 1-2-3-4-5-6-7-8-9-10

Diet: junk: junk food————semi-healthy————healthy

Greenhorn Group Workouts

Greenhorn Group Workout 1

Welcome to the Greenhorn Group Workout 1.

For this workout, you have 6 sets with 60 seconds of rest between each set.

Remember to focus on proper form throughout your sets.

Sets:

1. 19 sit-ups
2. 19 sit-ups
3. 19 sit-ups
4. 19 sit-ups
5. 19 sit-ups
6. 4 fundamental sit-ups with a 5 second descend.

If you completed this workout, head to Greenhorn Group Workout 2 for your next session. If not, stick with this one until you complete it.

Glasses of water drank today: 1-2-3-4-5-6-7-8-9-10

Hours of sleep last night: 1-2-3-4-5-6-7-8-9-10

Diet: junk: junk food————semi-healthy————healthy

Greenhorn Group Workout 2

Welcome to the Greenhorn Group Workout 2.

For this workout, you have 6 sets with 60 seconds of rest between each set.

Remember to focus on proper form throughout your sets.

Sets:

1. 20 sit-ups
2. 20 sit-ups
3. 20 sit-ups
4. 20 sit-ups
5. 20 sit-ups
6. 6 fundamental sit-ups with a 5 second descend.

If you completed this workout, head to Greenhorn Group Workout 3 for your next session. If not, stick with this one until you complete it.

Glasses of water drank today: 1-2-3-4-5-6-7-8-9-10

Hours of sleep last night: 1-2-3-4-5-6-7-8-9-10

Diet: junk: junk food————semi-healthy————healthy

Greenhorn Group Workout 3

Welcome to the Greenhorn Group Workout 3.

For this workout, you have 6 sets with 90 seconds of rest between each set.

Remember to focus on proper form throughout your sets.

Sets:

1. 23 sit-ups
2. 23 sit-ups
3. 23 sit-ups
4. 23 sit-ups
5. 23 sit-ups
6. Max out: perform as many sit-ups as you can.

Max reps: _____

If you completed this workout, head to Greenhorn Group Workout 4 for your next session. If not, stick with this one until you complete it.

Glasses of water drank today: 1-2-3-4-5-6-7-8-9-10

Hours of sleep last night: 1-2-3-4-5-6-7-8-9-10

Diet: junk: junk food—————semi-healthy—————healthy

Greenhorn Group Workout 4

Welcome to the Greenhorn Group Workout 4.

For this workout, you have 6 sets with 60 seconds of rest between each set.

Remember to focus on proper form throughout your sets.

Sets:

1. 25 sit-ups
2. 25 sit-ups
3. 25 sit-ups
4. 25 sit-ups
5. 25 sit-ups
6. 7 fundamental sit-ups with a 5 second descend.

If you completed this workout, head to Greenhorn Group Workout 5 for your next session. If not, stick with this one until you complete it.

Glasses of water drank today: 1-2-3-4-5-6-7-8-9-10

Hours of sleep last night: 1-2-3-4-5-6-7-8-9-10

Diet: junk: junk food————semi-healthy————healthy

Greenhorn Group Workout 5

Welcome to the Greenhorn Group Workout 5.

For this workout, you have 6 sets with 60 seconds of rest between each set.

Remember to focus on proper form throughout your sets.

Sets:

1. 28 sit-ups
2. 28 sit-ups
3. 28 sit-ups
4. 28 sit-ups
5. 28 sit-ups
6. 8 fundamental sit-ups with a 5 second descend.

If you completed this workout, head to Greenhorn Group Workout 6 for your next session. If not, stick with this one until you complete it.

Glasses of water drank today: 1-2-3-4-5-6-7-8-9-10

Hours of sleep last night: 1-2-3-4-5-6-7-8-9-10

Diet: junk: junk food————semi-healthy————healthy

Greenhorn Group Workout 6

Welcome to the Greenhorn Group Workout 6.

For this workout, you have 6 sets with 90 seconds of rest between each set.

Remember to focus on proper form throughout your sets.

Sets:

1. 31 sit-ups
2. 31 sit-ups
3. 31 sit-ups
4. 31 sit-ups
5. 31 sit-ups
6. Max out: perform as many sit-ups as you can.

Max reps: _____

Since this is the end of a two-week period, it is time to redo your sit-up assessment to check your progress if you fully completed this workout.

Rest a day and give the assessment a go to see which Group you will be in next.

Glasses of water drank today: 1-2-3-4-5-6-7-8-9-10

Hours of sleep last night: 1-2-3-4-5-6-7-8-9-10

Diet: junk: junk food—————semi-healthy—————healthy

Cub Group Workouts

Cub Group Workout 1

Welcome to the Cub Group Workout 1.

For this workout, you have 6 sets with 60 seconds of rest between each set.

Remember to focus on proper form throughout your sets.

Sets:

1. 23 sit-ups
2. 23 sit-ups
3. 23 sit-ups
4. 23 sit-ups
5. 23 sit-ups
6. 2 fundamental sit-ups with a 10 second descend.

If you completed this workout, head to Cub Group Workout 2 for your next session. If not, stick with this one until you complete it.

Glasses of water drank today: 1-2-3-4-5-6-7-8-9-10

Hours of sleep last night: 1-2-3-4-5-6-7-8-9-10

Diet: junk: junk food————semi-healthy————healthy

Cub Group Workout 2

Welcome to the Cub Group Workout 2.

For this workout, you have 6 sets with 60 seconds of rest between each set.

Remember to focus on proper form throughout your sets.

Sets:

1. 25 sit-ups
2. 25 sit-ups
3. 25 sit-ups
4. 25 sit-ups
5. 25 sit-ups
6. 3 fundamental sit-ups with a 10 second descend.

If you completed this workout, head to Cub Group Workout 3 for your next session. If not, stick with this one until you complete it.

Glasses of water drank today: 1-2-3-4-5-6-7-8-9-10

Hours of sleep last night: 1-2-3-4-5-6-7-8-9-10

Diet: junk: junk food————semi-healthy————healthy

Cub Group Workout 3

Welcome to the Cub Group Workout 3.

For this workout, you have 6 sets with 90 seconds of rest between each set.

Remember to focus on proper form throughout your sets.

Sets:

1. 28 sit-ups
2. 28 sit-ups
3. 28 sit-ups
4. 28 sit-ups
5. 28 sit-ups
6. Max out: perform as many sit-ups as you can.

Max reps: _____

If you completed this workout, head to Cub Group Workout 4 for your next session. If not, stick with this one until you complete it.

Glasses of water drank today: 1-2-3-4-5-6-7-8-9-10

Hours of sleep last night: 1-2-3-4-5-6-7-8-9-10

Diet: junk: junk food—————semi-healthy—————healthy

Cub Group Workout 4

Welcome to the Cub Group Workout 4.

For this workout, you have 6 sets with 60 seconds of rest between each set.

Remember to focus on proper form throughout your sets.

Sets:

1. 31 sit-ups
2. 31 sit-ups
3. 31 sit-ups
4. 31 sit-ups
5. 31 sit-ups
6. 4 fundamental sit-ups with a 10 second descend.

If you completed this workout, head to Cub Group Workout 5 for your next session. If not, stick with this one until you complete it.

Glasses of water drank today: 1-2-3-4-5-6-7-8-9-10

Hours of sleep last night: 1-2-3-4-5-6-7-8-9-10

Diet: junk: junk food————semi-healthy————healthy

Cub Group Workout 5

Welcome to the Cub Group Workout 5.

For this workout, you have 6 sets with 60 seconds of rest between each set.

Remember to focus on proper form throughout your sets.

Sets:

1. 34 sit-ups
2. 34 sit-ups
3. 34 sit-ups
4. 34 sit-ups
5. 34 sit-ups
6. 4 fundamental sit-ups with a 10 second descend.

If you completed this workout, head to Cub Group Workout 6 for your next session. If not, stick with this one until you complete it.

Glasses of water drank today: 1-2-3-4-5-6-7-8-9-10

Hours of sleep last night: 1-2-3-4-5-6-7-8-9-10

Diet: junk: junk food—————semi-healthy—————healthy

Cub Group Workout 6

Welcome to the Cub Group Workout 6.

For this workout, you have 6 sets with 90 seconds of rest between each set.

Remember to focus on proper form throughout your sets.

Sets:

1. 37 sit-ups
2. 37 sit-ups
3. 37 sit-ups
4. 37 sit-ups
5. 37 sit-ups
6. Max out: perform as many sit-ups as you can.

Max reps: _____

Since this is the end of a two-week period, it is time to redo your sit-up assessment to check your progress if you fully completed this workout.

Rest a day and give the assessment a go to see which Group you will be in next.

Glasses of water drank today: 1-2-3-4-5-6-7-8-9-10

Hours of sleep last night: 1-2-3-4-5-6-7-8-9-10

Diet: junk: junk food—————semi-healthy—————healthy

Rookie Group Workouts

Rookie Group Workout 1

Welcome to the Rookie Group Workout 1.

For this workout, you have 6 sets with 60 seconds of rest between each set.

Remember to focus on proper form throughout your sets.

Sets:

1. 28 sit-ups
2. 28 sit-ups
3. 28 sit-ups
4. 28 sit-ups
5. 28 sit-ups
6. 4 fundamental sit-ups with a 10 second descend.

If you completed this workout, head to Cub Group Workout 2 for your next session. If not, stick with this one until you complete it.

Glasses of water drank today: 1-2-3-4-5-6-7-8-9-10

Hours of sleep last night: 1-2-3-4-5-6-7-8-9-10

Diet: junk: junk food————semi-healthy————healthy

Rookie Group Workout 2

Welcome to the Rookie Group Workout 2.

For this workout, you have 6 sets with 60 seconds of rest between each set.

Remember to focus on proper form throughout your sets.

Sets:

1. 31 sit-ups
2. 31 sit-ups
3. 31 sit-ups
4. 31 sit-ups
5. 31 sit-ups
6. 4 fundamental sit-ups with a 10 second descend.

If you completed this workout, head to Rookie Group Workout 3 for your next session. If not, stick with this one until you complete it.

Glasses of water drank today: 1-2-3-4-5-6-7-8-9-10

Hours of sleep last night: 1-2-3-4-5-6-7-8-9-10

Diet: junk: junk food—————semi-healthy—————healthy

Rookie Group Workout 3

Welcome to the Rookie Group Workout 3.

For this workout, you have 6 sets with 90 seconds of rest between each set.

Remember to focus on proper form throughout your sets.

Sets:

1. 34 sit-ups
2. 34 sit-ups
3. 34 sit-ups
4. 34 sit-ups
5. 34 sit-ups
6. Max out: perform as many sit-ups as you can.

Max reps: _____

If you completed this workout, head to Rookie Group Workout 4 for your next session. If not, stick with this one until you complete it.

Glasses of water drank today: 1-2-3-4-5-6-7-8-9-10

Hours of sleep last night: 1-2-3-4-5-6-7-8-9-10

Diet: junk: junk food—————semi-healthy—————healthy

Rookie Group Workout 4

Welcome to the Rookie Group Workout 4.

For this workout, you have 6 sets with 60 seconds of rest between each set.

Remember to focus on proper form throughout your sets.

Sets:

1. 37 sit-ups
2. 37 sit-ups
3. 37 sit-ups
4. 37 sit-ups
5. 37 sit-ups
6. 6 fundamental sit-ups with a 10 second descend.

If you completed this workout, head to Rookie Group Workout 5 for your next session. If not, stick with this one until you complete it.

Glasses of water drank today: 1-2-3-4-5-6-7-8-9-10

Hours of sleep last night: 1-2-3-4-5-6-7-8-9-10

Diet: junk: junk food————semi-healthy————healthy

Rookie Group Workout 5

Welcome to the Rookie Group Workout 5.

For this workout, you have 6 sets with 60 seconds of rest between each set.

Remember to focus on proper form throughout your sets.

Sets:

1. 44 sit-ups
2. 44 sit-ups
3. 44 sit-ups
4. 44 sit-ups
5. 44 sit-ups
6. 7 fundamental sit-ups with a 10 second descend.

If you completed this workout, head to Rookie Group Workout 6 for your next session. If not, stick with this one until you complete it.

Glasses of water drank today: 1-2-3-4-5-6-7-8-9-10

Hours of sleep last night: 1-2-3-4-5-6-7-8-9-10

Diet: junk: junk food———––—semi-healthy———––—healthy

Rookie Group Workout 6

Welcome to the Rookie Group Workout 6.

For this workout, you have 6 sets with 90 seconds of rest between each set.

Remember to focus on proper form throughout your sets.

Sets:

1. 49 sit-ups
2. 49 sit-ups
3. 49 sit-ups
4. 49 sit-ups
5. 49 sit-ups
6. Max out: perform as many sit-ups as you can.

Max reps: _____

Since this is the end of a two-week period, it is time to redo your sit-up assessment to check your progress if you fully completed this workout.

Rest a day and give the assessment a go to see which Group you will be in next.

Glasses of water drank today: 1-2-3-4-5-6-7-8-9-10

Hours of sleep last night: 1-2-3-4-5-6-7-8-9-10

Diet: junk: junk food—————semi-healthy—————healthy

Pleb Group Workouts

Pleb Group Workout 1

Welcome to the Pleb Group Workout 1.

For this workout, you have 6 sets with 60 seconds of rest between each set.

Remember to focus on proper form throughout your sets.

Sets:

1. 34 sit-ups
2. 34 sit-ups
3. 34 sit-ups
4. 34 sit-ups
5. 34 sit-ups
6. 5 fundamental sit-ups with a 10 second descend.

If you completed this workout, head to Pleb Group Workout 2 for your next session. If not, stick with this one until you complete it.

Glasses of water drank today: 1-2-3-4-5-6-7-8-9-10

Hours of sleep last night: 1-2-3-4-5-6-7-8-9-10

Diet: junk: junk food————semi-healthy————healthy

Pleb Group Workout 2

Welcome to the Pleb Group Workout 2.

For this workout, you have 6 sets with 60 seconds of rest between each set.

Remember to focus on proper form throughout your sets.

Sets:

1. 38 sit-ups
2. 38 sit-ups
3. 38 sit-ups
4. 38 sit-ups
5. 38 sit-ups
6. 6 fundamental sit-ups with a 10 second descend.

If you completed this workout, head to Pleb Group Workout 3 for your next session. If not, stick with this one until you complete it.

Glasses of water drank today: 1-2-3-4-5-6-7-8-9-10

Hours of sleep last night: 1-2-3-4-5-6-7-8-9-10

Diet: junk: junk food————semi-healthy————healthy

Pleb Group Workout 3

Welcome to the Pleb Group Workout 3.

For this workout, you have 6 sets with 90 seconds of rest between each set.

Remember to focus on proper form throughout your sets.

Sets:

1. 42 sit-ups
2. 42 sit-ups
3. 42 sit-ups
4. 42 sit-ups
5. 42 sit-ups
6. Max out: perform as many sit-ups as you can.

Max reps: _____

If you completed this workout, head to Pleb Group Workout 4 for your next session. If not, stick with this one until you complete it.

Glasses of water drank today: 1-2-3-4-5-6-7-8-9-10

Hours of sleep last night: 1-2-3-4-5-6-7-8-9-10

Diet: junk: junk food—————semi-healthy—————healthy

Pleb Group Workout 4

Welcome to the Pleb Group Workout 4.

For this workout, you have 6 sets with 60 seconds of rest between each set.

Remember to focus on proper form throughout your sets.

Sets:

1. 45 sit-ups
2. 45 sit-ups
3. 45 sit-ups
4. 45 sit-ups
5. 45 sit-ups
6. 8 fundamental sit-ups with a 10 second descend.

If you completed this workout, head to Pleb Group Workout 5 for your next session. If not, stick with this one until you complete it.

Glasses of water drank today: 1-2-3-4-5-6-7-8-9-10

Hours of sleep last night: 1-2-3-4-5-6-7-8-9-10

Diet: junk: junk food————semi-healthy————healthy

Pleb Group Workout 5

Welcome to the Pleb Group Workout 5.

For this workout, you have 6 sets with 60 seconds of rest between each set.

Remember to focus on proper form throughout your sets.

Sets:

1. 53 sit-ups
2. 53 sit-ups
3. 53 sit-ups
4. 53 sit-ups
5. 53 sit-ups
6. 9 fundamental sit-ups with a 10 second descend.

If you completed this workout, head to Pleb Group Workout 6 for your next session. If not, stick with this one until you complete it.

Glasses of water drank today: 1-2-3-4-5-6-7-8-9-10

Hours of sleep last night: 1-2-3-4-5-6-7-8-9-10

Diet: junk: junk food————semi-healthy————healthy

Pleb Group Workout 6

Welcome to the Pleb Group Workout 6.

For this workout, you have 6 sets with 90 seconds of rest between each set.

Remember to focus on proper form throughout your sets.

Sets:

1. 61 sit-ups
2. 61 sit-ups
3. 61 sit-ups
4. 61 sit-ups
5. 61 sit-ups
6. Max out: perform as many sit-ups as you can.

Max reps: _____

Since this is the end of a two-week period, it is time to redo your sit-up assessment to check your progress if you fully completed this workout.

Rest a day and give the assessment a go to see which Group you will be in next.

Glasses of water drank today: 1-2-3-4-5-6-7-8-9-10

Hours of sleep last night: 1-2-3-4-5-6-7-8-9-10

Diet: junk: junk food————semi-healthy————healthy

Gorilla Group Workouts

Gorilla Group Workout 1

Welcome to the Gorilla Group Workout 1.

For this workout, you have 6 sets with 120 seconds of rest between each set.

Remember to focus on proper form throughout your sets.

Sets:

1. 42 sit-ups
2. 42 sit-ups
3. 42 sit-ups
4. 42 sit-ups
5. 42 sit-ups
6. 5 fundamental sit-ups with a 10 second descend.

If you completed this workout, head to Gorilla Group Workout 2 for your next session. If not, stick with this one until you complete it.

Glasses of water drank today: 1-2-3-4-5-6-7-8-9-10

Hours of sleep last night: 1-2-3-4-5-6-7-8-9-10

Diet: junk: junk food————semi-healthy————healthy

Gorilla Group Workout 2

Welcome to the Gorilla Group Workout 2.

For this workout, you have 9 sets with 90 seconds of rest between each set.

Remember to focus on proper form throughout your sets.

Sets:

1. 28 sit-ups
2. 28 sit-ups
3. 28 sit-ups
4. 28 sit-ups
5. 28 sit-ups
6. 28 sit-ups
7. 28 sit-ups
8. 28 sit-ups
9. 6 fundamental sit-ups with a 10 second descend.

If you completed this workout, head to Gorilla Group Workout 3 for your next session. If not, stick with this one until you complete it.

Glasses of water drank today: 1-2-3-4-5-6-7-8-9-10

Hours of sleep last night: 1-2-3-4-5-6-7-8-9-10

Diet: junk: junk food—————semi-healthy—————healthy

Gorilla Group Workout 3

Welcome to the Gorilla Group Workout 3.

For this workout, you have 9 sets with 90 seconds of rest between each set.

Remember to focus on proper form throughout your sets.

Sets:

1. 30 sit-ups
2. 30 sit-ups
3. 30 sit-ups
4. 30 sit-ups
5. 30 sit-ups
6. 30 sit-ups
7. 30 sit-ups
8. 30 sit-ups
9. Max out: perform as many sit-ups as you can.

Max reps: _____

If you completed this workout, head to Gorilla Group Workout 4 for your next session. If not, stick with this one until you complete it.

Glasses of water drank today: 1-2-3-4-5-6-7-8-9-10

Hours of sleep last night: 1-2-3-4-5-6-7-8-9-10

Diet: junk: junk food—————semi-healthy—————healthy

Gorilla Group Workout 4

Welcome to the Gorilla Group Workout 4.

For this workout, you have 6 sets with 120 seconds of rest between each set.

Remember to focus on proper form throughout your sets.

Sets:

1. 61 sit-ups
2. 61 sit-ups
3. 61 sit-ups
4. 61 sit-ups
5. 61 sit-ups
6. 10 fundamental sit-ups with a 10 second descend.

If you completed this workout, head to Gorilla Group Workout 5 for your next session. If not, stick with this one until you complete it.

Glasses of water drank today: 1-2-3-4-5-6-7-8-9-10

Hours of sleep last night: 1-2-3-4-5-6-7-8-9-10

Diet: junk: junk food—————semi-healthy—————healthy

Gorilla Group Workout 5

Welcome to the Gorilla Group Workout 5.

For this workout, you have 10 sets with 90 seconds of rest between each set.

Remember to focus on proper form throughout your sets.

Sets:

1. 35 sit-ups
2. 35 sit-ups
3. 35 sit-ups
4. 35 sit-ups
5. 35 sit-ups
6. 35 sit-ups
7. 35 sit-ups
8. 35 sit-ups
9. 35 sit-ups
10. 11 fundamental sit-ups with a 10 second descend.

If you completed this workout, head to Gorilla Group Workout 6 for your next session. If not, stick with this one until you complete it.

Glasses of water drank today: 1-2-3-4-5-6-7-8-9-10

Hours of sleep last night: 1-2-3-4-5-6-7-8-9-10

Diet: junk: junk food————semi-healthy————healthy

Gorilla Group Workout 6

Welcome to the Gorilla Group Workout 6.

For this workout, you have 10 sets with 90 seconds of rest between each set.

Remember to focus on proper form throughout your sets.

Sets:

1. 37 sit-ups
2. 37 sit-ups
3. 37 sit-ups
4. 37 sit-ups
5. 37 sit-ups
6. 37 sit-ups
7. 37 sit-ups
8. 37 sit-ups
9. 37 sit-ups
10. Max out: perform as many sit-ups as you can.

Max reps: _____

Since this is the end of a two-week period, it is time to redo your sit-up assessment to check your progress if you fully completed this workout.

Rest a day and give the assessment a go to see which Group you will be in next.

Glasses of water drank today: 1-2-3-4-5-6-7-8-9-10

Hours of sleep last night: 1-2-3-4-5-6-7-8-9-10

Diet: junk: junk food————semi-healthy————healthy

Viking Group Workouts

Viking Group Workout 1

Welcome to the Viking Group Workout 1.

For this workout, you have 6 sets with 120 seconds of rest between each set.

Remember to focus on proper form throughout your sets.

Sets:

1. 56 sit-ups
2. 56 sit-ups
3. 56 sit-ups
4. 56 sit-ups
5. 56 sit-ups
6. 8 fundamental sit-ups with a 10 second descend.

If you completed this workout, head to Viking Group Workout 2 for your next session. If not, stick with this one until you complete it.

Glasses of water drank today: 1-2-3-4-5-6-7-8-9-10

Hours of sleep last night: 1-2-3-4-5-6-7-8-9-10

Diet: junk: junk food—————semi-healthy—————healthy

Viking Group Workout 2

Welcome to the Viking Group Workout 2.

For this workout, you have 9 sets with 90 seconds of rest between each set.

Remember to focus on proper form throughout your sets.

Sets:

1. 35 sit-ups
2. 35 sit-ups
3. 35 sit-ups
4. 35 sit-ups
5. 35 sit-ups
6. 35 sit-ups
7. 35 sit-ups
8. 35 sit-ups
9. 10 fundamental sit-ups with a 10 second descend.

If you completed this workout, head to Viking Group Workout 3 for your next session. If not, stick with this one until you complete it.

Glasses of water drank today: 1-2-3-4-5-6-7-8-9-10

Hours of sleep last night: 1-2-3-4-5-6-7-8-9-10

Diet: junk: junk food—————semi-healthy—————healthy

Viking Group Workout 3

Welcome to the Viking Group Workout 3.

For this workout, you have 9 sets with 90 seconds of rest between each set.

Remember to focus on proper form throughout your sets.

Sets:

1. 37 sit-ups
2. 37 sit-ups
3. 37 sit-ups
4. 37 sit-ups
5. 37 sit-ups
6. 37 sit-ups
7. 37 sit-ups
8. 37 sit-ups
9. Max out: perform as many sit-ups as you can.

Max reps: _____

If you completed this workout, head to Viking Group Workout 4 for your next session. If not, stick with this one until you complete it.

Glasses of water drank today: 1-2-3-4-5-6-7-8-9-10

Hours of sleep last night: 1-2-3-4-5-6-7-8-9-10

Diet: junk: junk food————semi-healthy————healthy

Viking Group Workout 4

Welcome to the Viking Group Workout 4.

For this workout, you have 6 sets with 120 seconds of rest between each set.

Remember to focus on proper form throughout your sets.

Sets:

1. 70 sit-ups
2. 70 sit-ups
3. 70 sit-ups
4. 70 sit-ups
5. 70 sit-ups
6. 12 fundamental sit-ups with a 10 second descend.

If you completed this workout, head to Viking Group Workout 5 for your next session. If not, stick with this one until you complete it.

Glasses of water drank today: 1-2-3-4-5-6-7-8-9-10

Hours of sleep last night: 1-2-3-4-5-6-7-8-9-10

Diet: junk: junk food————semi-healthy————healthy

Viking Group Workout 5

Welcome to the Viking Group Workout 5.

For this workout, you have 10 sets with 90 seconds of rest between each set.

Remember to focus on proper form throughout your sets.

Sets:

1. 41 sit-ups
2. 41 sit-ups
3. 41 sit-ups
4. 41 sit-ups
5. 41 sit-ups
6. 41 sit-ups
7. 41 sit-ups
8. 41 sit-ups
9. 41 sit-ups
10. 13 fundamental sit-ups with a 10 second descend.

If you completed this workout, head to Viking Group Workout 6 for your next session. If not, stick with this one until you complete it.

Glasses of water drank today: 1-2-3-4-5-6-7-8-9-10

Hours of sleep last night: 1-2-3-4-5-6-7-8-9-10

Diet: junk: junk food————semi-healthy————healthy

Viking Group Workout 6

Welcome to the Viking Group Workout 6.

For this workout, you have 10 sets with 90 seconds of rest between each set.

Remember to focus on proper form throughout your sets.

Sets:

1. 48 sit-ups
2. 48 sit-ups
3. 48 sit-ups
4. 48 sit-ups
5. 48 sit-ups
6. 48 sit-ups
7. 48 sit-ups
8. 48 sit-ups
9. 48 sit-ups
10. Max out: perform as many sit-ups as you can.

Max reps: _____

Since this is the end of a two-week period, it is time to redo your sit-ups assessment to check your progress if you fully completed this workout.

Rest a day and give the assessment a go to see which Group you will be in next.

Glasses of water drank today: 1-2-3-4-5-6-7-8-9-10

Hours of sleep last night: 1-2-3-4-5-6-7-8-9-10

Diet: junk: junk food————semi-healthy————healthy

Elite Group Workouts

Elite Group Workout 1

Welcome to the Elite Group Workout 1.

For this workout, you have 6 sets with 120 seconds of rest between each set.

Remember to focus on proper form throughout your sets.

Sets:

1. 66 sit-ups
2. 66 sit-ups
3. 66 sit-ups
4. 66 sit-ups
5. 66 sit-ups
6. 10 fundamental sit-ups with a 10 second descend.

If you completed this workout, head to Elite Group Workout 2 for your next session. If not, stick with this one until you complete it.

Glasses of water drank today: 1-2-3-4-5-6-7-8-9-10

Hours of sleep last night: 1-2-3-4-5-6-7-8-9-10

Diet: junk: junk food————semi-healthy————healthy

Elite Group Workout 2

Welcome to the Elite Group Workout 2.

For this workout, you have 9 sets with 90 seconds of rest between each set.

Remember to focus on proper form throughout your sets.

Sets:

1. 30 sit-ups
2. 30 sit-ups
3. 30 sit-ups
4. 30 sit-ups
5. 30 sit-ups
6. 30 sit-ups
7. 30 sit-ups
8. 30 sit-ups
9. 11 fundamental sit-ups with a 10 second descend.

If you completed this workout, head to Elite Group Workout 3 for your next session. If not, stick with this one until you complete it.

Glasses of water drank today: 1-2-3-4-5-6-7-8-9-10

Hours of sleep last night: 1-2-3-4-5-6-7-8-9-10

Diet: junk: junk food————semi-healthy————healthy

Elite Group Workout 3

Welcome to the Elite Group Workout 3.

For this workout, you have 9 sets with 90 seconds of rest between each set.

Remember to focus on proper form throughout your sets.

Sets:

1. 43 sit-ups
2. 43 sit-ups
3. 43 sit-ups
4. 43 sit-ups
5. 43 sit-ups
6. 43 sit-ups
7. 43 sit-ups
8. 43 sit-ups
9. Max out: perform as many sit-ups as you can.

Max reps: _____

If you completed this workout, head to Elite Group Workout 4 for your next session. If not, stick with this one until you complete it.

Glasses of water drank today: 1-2-3-4-5-6-7-8-9-10

Hours of sleep last night: 1-2-3-4-5-6-7-8-9-10

Diet: junk: junk food————semi-healthy————healthy

Elite Group Workout 4

Welcome to the Elite Group Workout 4.

For this workout, you have 6 sets with 120 seconds of rest between each set.

Remember to focus on proper form throughout your sets.

Sets:

1. 83 sit-ups
2. 83 sit-ups
3. 83 sit-ups
4. 83 sit-ups
5. 83 sit-ups
6. 14 fundamental sit-ups with a 10 second descend.

If you completed this workout, head to Elite Group Workout 5 for your next session. If not, stick with this one until you complete it.

Glasses of water drank today: 1-2-3-4-5-6-7-8-9-10

Hours of sleep last night: 1-2-3-4-5-6-7-8-9-10

Diet: junk: junk food————semi-healthy————healthy

Elite Group Workout 5

Welcome to the Elite Group Workout 5.

For this workout, you have 10 sets with 90 seconds of rest between each set.

Remember to focus on proper form throughout your sets.

Sets:

1. 48 sit-ups
2. 48 sit-ups
3. 48 sit-ups
4. 48 sit-ups
5. 48 sit-ups
6. 48 sit-ups
7. 48 sit-ups
8. 48 sit-ups
9. 48 sit-ups
10. 15 fundamental sit-ups with a 10 second descend.

If you completed this workout, head to Elite Group Workout 6 for your next session. If not, stick with this one until you complete it.

Glasses of water drank today: 1-2-3-4-5-6-7-8-9-10

Hours of sleep last night: 1-2-3-4-5-6-7-8-9-10

Diet: junk: junk food————semi-healthy————healthy

Elite Group Workout 6

Welcome to the Elite Group Workout 6.

For this workout, you have 10 sets with 90 seconds of rest between each set.

Remember to focus on proper form throughout your sets.

Sets:

1. 54 sit-ups
2. 54 sit-ups
3. 54 sit-ups
4. 54 sit-ups
5. 54 sit-ups
6. 54 sit-ups
7. 54 sit-ups
8. 54 sit-ups
9. 54 sit-ups
10. Max out: perform as many sit-ups as you can.

Max reps: _____

Since this is the end of a two-week period, it is time to redo your sit-up assessment to check your progress if you fully completed this workout.

Rest a day and give the assessment a go to see which Group you will be in next.

Glasses of water drank today: 1-2-3-4-5-6-7-8-9-10

Hours of sleep last night: 1-2-3-4-5-6-7-8-9-10

Diet: junk: junk food—————semi-healthy—————healthy

Commando Group Workouts

Commando Group Workout 1

Welcome to the Commando Group Workout 1.

For this workout, you have 6 sets with 120 seconds of rest between each set.

Remember to focus on proper form throughout your sets.

Sets:

1. 70 sit-ups
2. 70 sit-ups
3. 70 sit-ups
4. 70 sit-ups
5. 70 sit-ups
6. 11 fundamental sit-ups with a 10 second descend.

If you completed this workout, head to Commando Group Workout 2 for your next session. If not, stick with this one until you complete it.

Glasses of water drank today: 1-2-3-4-5-6-7-8-9-10

Hours of sleep last night: 1-2-3-4-5-6-7-8-9-10

Diet: junk: junk food—————semi-healthy—————healthy

Commando Group Workout 2

Welcome to the Commando Group Workout 2.

For this workout, you have 10 sets with 90 seconds of rest between each set.

Remember to focus on proper form throughout your sets.

Sets:

1. 31 sit-ups
2. 31 sit-ups
3. 31 sit-ups
4. 31 sit-ups
5. 31 sit-ups
6. 31 sit-ups
7. 31 sit-ups
8. 31 sit-ups
9. 31 sit-ups
10. 12 fundamental sit-ups with a 10 second descend.

If you completed this workout, head to Commando Group Workout 3 for your next session. If not, stick with this one until you complete it.

Glasses of water drank today: 1-2-3-4-5-6-7-8-9-10

Hours of sleep last night: 1-2-3-4-5-6-7-8-9-10

Diet: junk: junk food————semi-healthy————healthy

Commando Group Workout 3

Welcome to the Commando Group Workout 3.

For this workout, you have 10 sets with 90 seconds of rest between each set.

Remember to focus on proper form throughout your sets.

Sets:

1. 46 sit-ups
2. 46 sit-ups
3. 46 sit-ups
4. 46 sit-ups
5. 46 sit-ups
6. 46 sit-ups
7. 46 sit-ups
8. 46 sit-ups
9. 46 sit-ups
10. Max out: perform as many sit-ups as you can.

Max reps: _____

If you completed this workout, head to Commando Group Workout 4 for your next session. If not, stick with this one until you complete it.

Glasses of water drank today: 1-2-3-4-5-6-7-8-9-10

Hours of sleep last night: 1-2-3-4-5-6-7-8-9-10

Diet: junk: junk food————semi-healthy————healthy

Commando Group Workout 4

Welcome to the Commando Group Workout 4.

For this workout, you have 6 sets with 120 seconds of rest between each set.

Remember to focus on proper form throughout your sets.

Sets:

1. 86 sit-ups
2. 86 sit-ups
3. 86 sit-ups
4. 86 sit-ups
5. 86 sit-ups
6. 13 fundamental sit-ups with a 10 second descend.

If you completed this workout, head to Commando Group Workout 5 for your next session. If not, stick with this one until you complete it.

Glasses of water drank today: 1-2-3-4-5-6-7-8-9-10

Hours of sleep last night: 1-2-3-4-5-6-7-8-9-10

Diet: junk: junk food—————semi-healthy—————healthy

Commando Group Workout 5

Welcome to the Commando Group Workout 5.

For this workout, you have 10 sets with 90 seconds of rest between each set.

Remember to focus on proper form throughout your sets.

Sets:

1. 52 sit-ups
2. 52 sit-ups
3. 52 sit-ups
4. 52 sit-ups
5. 52 sit-ups
6. 52 sit-ups
7. 52 sit-ups
8. 52 sit-ups
9. 52 sit-ups
10. 14 fundamental sit-ups with a 10 second descend.

If you completed this workout, head to Commando Group Workout 6 for your next session. If not, stick with this one until you complete it.

Glasses of water drank today: 1-2-3-4-5-6-7-8-9-10

Hours of sleep last night: 1-2-3-4-5-6-7-8-9-10

Diet: junk: junk food—————semi-healthy—————healthy

Commando Group Workout 6

Welcome to the Commando Group Workout 6.

For this workout, you have 10 sets with 90 seconds of rest between each set.

Remember to focus on proper form throughout your sets.

Sets:

1. 58 sit-ups
2. 58 sit-ups
3. 58 sit-ups
4. 58 sit-ups
5. 58 sit-ups
6. 58 sit-ups
7. 58 sit-ups
8. 58 sit-ups
9. 58 sit-ups
10. Max out: perform as many sit-ups as you can.

Max reps: _____

If you completed this workout, you have earned the right to attempt hitting 200 consecutive sit-ups. Take a few days off to fully recover and take a shot

at hitting your goal.

You got this.

Glasses of water drank today: 1-2-3-4-5-6-7-8-9-10

Hours of sleep last night: 1-2-3-4-5-6-7-8-9-10

Diet: junk: junk food————semi-healthy————healthy

Veteran Group Workouts

Veteran Group Workout 1

Welcome to the Veteran Group Workout 1.

For this workout, you have 6 sets with 120 seconds of rest between each set.

Remember to focus on proper form throughout your sets.

Sets:

1. 86 sit-ups
2. 86 sit-ups
3. 86 sit-ups
4. 86 sit-ups
5. 86 sit-ups
6. 14 fundamental sit-ups with a 10 second descend.

If you completed this workout, head to Veteran Group Workout 2 for your next session. If not, stick with this one until you complete it.

Glasses of water drank today: 1-2-3-4-5-6-7-8-9-10

Hours of sleep last night: 1-2-3-4-5-6-7-8-9-10

Diet: junk: junk food————semi-healthy————healthy

Veteran Group Workout 2

Welcome to the Veteran Group Workout 2.

For this workout, you have 10 sets with 90 seconds of rest between each set.

Remember to focus on proper form throughout your sets.

Sets:

1. 45 sit-ups
2. 45 sit-ups
3. 45 sit-ups
4. 45 sit-ups
5. 45 sit-ups
6. 45 sit-ups
7. 45 sit-ups
8. 45 sit-ups
9. 45 sit-ups
10. 15 fundamental sit-ups with a 10 second descend.

If you completed this workout, head to Veteran Group Workout 3 for your next session. If not, stick with this one until you complete it.

Glasses of water drank today: 1-2-3-4-5-6-7-8-9-10

Hours of sleep last night: 1-2-3-4-5-6-7-8-9-10

Diet: junk: junk food—————semi-healthy—————healthy

Veteran Group Workout 3

Welcome to the Veteran Group Workout 3.

For this workout, you have 10 sets with 90 seconds of rest between each set.

Remember to focus on proper form throughout your sets.

Sets:

1. 52 sit-ups
2. 52 sit-ups
3. 52 sit-ups
4. 52 sit-ups
5. 52 sit-ups
6. 52 sit-ups
7. 52 sit-ups
8. 52 sit-ups
9. 52 sit-ups
10. Max out: perform as many sit-ups as you can.

Max reps: _____

If you completed this workout, head to Veteran Group Workout 4 for your next session. If not, stick with this one until you complete it.

Glasses of water drank today: 1-2-3-4-5-6-7-8-9-10

Hours of sleep last night: 1-2-3-4-5-6-7-8-9-10

Diet: junk: junk food—————semi-healthy—————healthy

Veteran Group Workout 4

Welcome to the Veteran Group Workout 4.

For this workout, you have 6 sets with 120 seconds of rest between each set.

Remember to focus on proper form throughout your sets.

Sets:

1. 106 sit-ups
2. 106 sit-ups
3. 106 sit-ups
4. 106 sit-ups
5. 106 sit-ups
6. 16 fundamental sit-ups with a 10 second descend.

If you completed this workout, head to Veteran Group Workout 5 for your next session. If not, stick with this one until you complete it.

Glasses of water drank today: 1-2-3-4-5-6-7-8-9-10

Hours of sleep last night: 1-2-3-4-5-6-7-8-9-10

Diet: junk: junk food————semi-healthy————healthy

Veteran Group Workout 5

Welcome to the Veteran Group Workout 5.

For this workout, you have 10 sets with 90 seconds of rest between each set.

Remember to focus on proper form throughout your sets.

Sets:

1. 58 sit-ups
2. 58 sit-ups
3. 58 sit-ups
4. 58 sit-ups
5. 58 sit-ups
6. 58 sit-ups
7. 58 sit-ups
8. 58 sit-ups
9. 58 sit-ups
10. 17 fundamental sit-ups with a 10 second descend.

If you completed this workout, head to Veteran Group Workout 6 for your next session. If not, stick with this one until you complete it.

Glasses of water drank today: 1-2-3-4-5-6-7-8-9-10

Hours of sleep last night: 1-2-3-4-5-6-7-8-9-10

Diet: junk: junk food————semi-healthy————healthy

Veteran Group Workout 6

Welcome to the Veteran Group Workout 6.

For this workout, you have 10 sets with 90 seconds of rest between each set.

Remember to focus on proper form throughout your sets.

Sets:

1. 66 sit-ups
2. 66 sit-ups
3. 66 sit-ups
4. 66 sit-ups
5. 66 sit-ups
6. 66 sit-ups
7. 66 sit-ups
8. 66 sit-ups
9. 66 sit-ups
10. Max out: perform as many sit-ups as you can.

Max reps: _____

If you completed this workout, you have earned the right to attempt hitting 200 consecutive sit-ups. Take a few days off to fully recover and take a shot

at hitting your goal.

You got this.

Glasses of water drank today: 1-2-3-4-5-6-7-8-9-10

Hours of sleep last night: 1-2-3-4-5-6-7-8-9-10

Diet: junk: junk food————semi-healthy————healthy

Nuclear Group Workouts

Nuclear Group Workout 1

Welcome to the Nuclear Group Workout 1.

For this workout, you have 6 sets with 120 seconds of rest between each set.

Remember to focus on proper form throughout your sets.

Sets:

1. 99 sit-ups
2. 99 sit-ups
3. 99 sit-ups
4. 99 sit-ups
5. 99 sit-ups
6. 15 fundamental sit-ups with a 10 second descend.

If you completed this workout, head to Nuclear Group Workout 2 for your next session. If not, stick with this one until you complete it.

Glasses of water drank today: 1-2-3-4-5-6-7-8-9-10

Hours of sleep last night: 1-2-3-4-5-6-7-8-9-10

Diet: junk: junk food————semi-healthy————healthy

Nuclear Group Workout 2

Welcome to the Nuclear Group Workout 2.

For this workout, you have 10 sets with 90 seconds of rest between each set.

Remember to focus on proper form throughout your sets.

Sets:

1. 52 sit-ups
2. 52 sit-ups
3. 52 sit-ups
4. 52 sit-ups
5. 52 sit-ups
6. 52 sit-ups
7. 52 sit-ups
8. 52 sit-ups
9. 52 sit-ups
10. 16 fundamental sit-ups with a 10 second descend.

If you completed this workout, head to Nuclear Group Workout 3 for your next session. If not, stick with this one until you complete it.

Glasses of water drank today: 1-2-3-4-5-6-7-8-9-10

Hours of sleep last night: 1-2-3-4-5-6-7-8-9-10

Diet: junk: junk food—————semi-healthy—————healthy

Nuclear Group Workout 3

Welcome to the Nuclear Group Workout 3.

For this workout, you have 10 sets with 90 seconds of rest between each set.

Remember to focus on proper form throughout your sets.

Sets:

1. 58 sit-ups
2. 58 sit-ups
3. 58 sit-ups
4. 58 sit-ups
5. 58 sit-ups
6. 58 sit-ups
7. 58 sit-ups
8. 58 sit-ups
9. 58 sit-ups
10. Max out: perform as many sit-ups as you can.

Max reps: _____

If you completed this workout, head to Nuclear Group Workout 4 for your next session. If not, stick with this one until you complete it.

Glasses of water drank today: 1-2-3-4-5-6-7-8-9-10

Hours of sleep last night: 1-2-3-4-5-6-7-8-9-10

Diet: junk: junk food—————semi-healthy—————healthy

Nuclear Group Workout 4

Welcome to the Nuclear Group Workout 4.

For this workout, you have 6 sets with 120 seconds of rest between each set.

Remember to focus on proper form throughout your sets.

Sets:

1. 109 sit-ups
2. 109 sit-ups
3. 109 sit-ups
4. 109 sit-ups
5. 109 sit-ups
6. 17 fundamental sit-ups with a 10 second descend.

If you completed this workout, head to Nuclear Group Workout 5 for your next session. If not, stick with this one until you complete it.

Glasses of water drank today: 1-2-3-4-5-6-7-8-9-10

Hours of sleep last night: 1-2-3-4-5-6-7-8-9-10

Diet: junk: junk food————semi-healthy————healthy

Nuclear Group Workout 5

Welcome to the Nuclear Group Workout 5.

For this workout, you have 10 sets with 90 seconds of rest between each set.

Remember to focus on proper form throughout your sets.

Sets:

1. 66 sit-ups
2. 66 sit-ups
3. 66 sit-ups
4. 66 sit-ups
5. 66 sit-ups
6. 66 sit-ups
7. 66 sit-ups
8. 66 sit-ups
9. 66 sit-ups
10. 18 fundamental sit-ups with a 10 second descend.

If you completed this workout, head to Nuclear Group Workout 6 for your next session. If not, stick with this one until you complete it.

Glasses of water drank today: 1-2-3-4-5-6-7-8-9-10

Hours of sleep last night: 1-2-3-4-5-6-7-8-9-10

Diet: junk: junk food—————semi-healthy—————healthy

Nuclear Group Workout 6

Welcome to the Nuclear Group Workout 6.

For this workout, you have 10 sets with 90 seconds of rest between each set.

Remember to focus on proper form throughout your sets.

Sets:

1. 70 sit-ups
2. 70 sit-ups
3. 70 sit-ups
4. 70 sit-ups
5. 70 sit-ups
6. 70 sit-ups
7. 70 sit-ups
8. 70 sit-ups
9. 70 sit-ups
10. Max out: perform as many sit-ups as you can.

Max reps: _____

If you completed this workout, you have earned the right to attempt hitting 200 consecutive sit-ups. Take a few days off to fully recover and take a shot

at hitting your goal.

You got this.

Glasses of water drank today: 1-2-3-4-5-6-7-8-9-10

Hours of sleep last night: 1-2-3-4-5-6-7-8-9-10

Diet: junk: junk food————semi-healthy————healthy

Attempting 200 Consecutive Sit-ups

If you are here, that means you have completed either the Commando, Veteran, or Nuclear Group Workouts and have earned the right to attempt nailing down 200 consecutive sit-ups.

This goal is well within your grasp and all you have to do is take it.

As you begin to warm up to crush this, I would like to ask a favor.

I am going to be greedy for a minute here and ask you to leave a review for the book.

Reviews are a pain to get but it will only take a minute or two to leave one.

Scan this QR which will take you straight to the book's page on Amazon.

Scroll down and click the 'leave a customer review' button, select your star rating, leave a few words, and that is it!

It is that simple!

Once that is done, get ready to crush this.

Get psyched for what is about to happen.

Give it everything you have got to knock out as many correct sit-ups without stopping.

Once you are done, come back.

* * *

If you nailed 200 or more, awesome.

That is incredible. Time to knock that off your bucket list.

If you did not quite get it, no worries. Not everyone gets it on the first try.

Use this number as your new assessment number and get back at it!

Cheers.

Conclusion:

I just want to thank you for making your way through this program and the book. You have bettered yourself for it.

I hope you have challenged yourself and I hope you tasted victory by reaching 200 consecutive sit-ups.

If you are hungry for more challenges, we have got plenty more where this came from.

And if you have enjoyed this book, do take a second to leave a review.

Until next time.

Cheers.

www.ingramcontent.com/pod-product-compliance
Lightning Source LLC
Chambersburg PA
CBHW022058020426
42335CB00012B/742